A Better Normal for Libido

Your Guide to Rediscovering Intimacy After
Cancer

Tess Devèze

CONTENTS

WHY I WROTE THIS BOOK

Hello! It's so wonderful to meet you. I'm Tess.

I thought before we get into the more 'intimate' details, I'd introduce myself and let you know what this book is about.

I was diagnosed with stage-three breast cancer in 2018, at the age of 36. At the time of my diagnosis, I'd been working in the sexuality sector for years. Over the years since my cancer diagnosis and endless treatments, only twice did a healthcare professional voluntarily bring up the topic of sexuality and only one booklet was recommended to me (which I had to go and find myself). The lack of information and support on this topic, both during and after treatments, was painfully noticeable.

Why aren't more resources available? Why are we so afraid to talk about this essential aspect of our lives?

First and foremost, I'm an occupational therapist (OT). What's an OT, I hear you ask? We are functional therapists and use specific approaches to promote independence and participation in 'occupations' which are any kind of meaningful life activity that occupies us. OT's help you do the day-to-day activities that you need and want to do, as best you can. This may include self-care tasks (shower, dressing, toileting), work related (vocational) tasks, social or community activities…and may also include sex!

My clinical experience is mostly in sexuality - during and after cancer treatments, brain-injury, neurological conditions, and those living with disability. Before moving solely to sexuality for people with cancer, disability and chronic illness, most of my work was in private and public hospitals across Australia, working in neurological rehabilitation. I love neuroscience, and most of my work is based on neurological concepts.

Other than having cancer and being a sexuality OT, I also work with sexuality and self-development pioneers 'Curious Creatures', based in Melbourne Australia. I've facilitated hundreds of workshops online and face to face for nearing a decade, teaching consent, better intimacy and communication skills. I've seen thousands of people's lives change through a deeper understanding of sexual intimacy.

Lastly, I've also studied somatic sexological bodywork at the Institute of Somatic Sexology. This training has given me a deeper understanding of how libido, pleasure, arousal and orgasmicity (cool word huh?) work on a physiological, neurological, and psychological level. These learnings form an essential part of this book.

Even with all my training, I've struggled. If you're struggling too, you're not alone (even if it doesn't get spoken about).

But it's not just about me. The contents of this book are also guided by you. I have a Facebook group 'Intimacy and Cancer' with thousands of people - all cancers, all genders - from over 49 countries, who share and support each other on this topic. My one-on-one clients have also been a huge source of learning, generously sharing their experiences.

It's been almost two years since releasing 'A Better Normal; Your Guide to Rediscovering Intimacy After Cancer', and the positive feedback I have personally been receiving from readers has been at times overwhelming. I am humbled, amazed and inspired by the impact and influence this book has had for those out there suffering.

But cancer treatments are *haaaaaard*, and so is reading! I wanted to know how I could reach more people, change more lives for the better through the contents in this book. In answer to that question, I've created the 'A Better Normal' mini-book *series*. It's a number of bite-sized treatment or side-effect specific mini-books, to help cancer patients and their loved ones maintain and grow connection, intimacy and sexuality. Each mini-book is created from the information in 'A Better Normal; Your Guide to Rediscovering Intimacy After Cancer', but broken down into simple, easy-to-read guides relative to your very specific needs, because often during and after treatments committing to a 300-page book feels overwhelming or is simply not possible.

Books in the 'A Better Normal' mini-book series are:

- 'A Better Normal for **Libido**; Your Guide to Rediscovering Intimacy After Cancer'
- 'A Better Normal for **Vaginal Dryness & Pain**; Your Guide to Rediscovering Intimacy After Cancer'
- 'A Better Normal for **Body Confidence**; Your Guide to Rediscovering Intimacy After Cancer'
- 'A Better Normal for **Chemotherapy**; Your Guide to Rediscovering Intimacy After Cancer'
- 'A Better Normal for **Hormone Therapy**; Your Guide to Rediscovering Intimacy After Cancer'
- 'A Better Normal for **Fatigue**; Your Guide to Rediscovering Intimacy After Cancer'

- 'A Better Normal for **Changes In Erection**; Your Guide to Rediscovering Intimacy After Cancer'
- 'A Better Normal for **Radiotherapy**; Your Guide to Rediscovering Intimacy After Cancer'
- 'A Better Normal for **Pain**; Your Guide to Rediscovering Intimacy After Cancer'

Or if you're after all of the above information (and more) in one place, the all-in-one book 'A Better Normal; Your Guide to Rediscovering Intimacy After Cancer' has everything you need.

If you end up with several mini-books in the series, that's pretty normal, as we don't have only one side-effect (geez, wouldn't that be nice!), and we can have the same side-effect from more than one treatment (like fatigue, or changes in libido). Cancer treatments impact us differently, which is why some books in this series are side-effect specific, and others treatment specific. So you can pick and choose what is most relevant for you and where you're at. You'll also notice that some mini-books have repeated information in them. That's because some information is essential and helpful, regardless of what your side-effect or treatment is (like the communication tips, or ways to gently reconnect with yourself or a partner).

The most important thing you can learn from this book is that you're not alone and you're not broken. There's nothing wrong with you if you're struggling. It's normal to find this situation tough. This isn't one-size-fits-all advice. All bodies are unique, every relationship is different, and everyone experiences relationships, connection, pleasure and desire in their own way. You're the expert on you! Just as cancer is different for everyone, so are the connections we have with ourselves and those around us.

Lastly, this book is for all human beings, regardless of gender, lifestyle, orientation, ability, ethnicity, age, or relationship dynamic. Although every person with cancer is unique, we have one thing in common: no matter who we are or what we are going through, we're all worthy of love and connection.

Now, let's get started on making your 'new normal', a 'better normal'.

1. KEY TERMS EXPLAINED

Sexuality vs sex

The word 'sexuality' is an umbrella term which yes includes the functional activity of sex, but also includes relationships, connections, affection, dating, pleasure and our overall well-being. Sexuality can be greatly affected due to cancer, but it doesn't necessarily have to stop altogether. As a sexuality educator and clinician, I know how important sexuality, connection and intimacy is to our quality of life, our resilience and coping. What could be more important!

'Sex' in this book refers to the act, or the activity you engage in with yourself and/others, and is one of the most diverse and most adaptable functional activities I can think of. Yet today, it's still one of the most under-addressed topics in clinical settings. This is something I aim to change.

I also want us all to be on the same page in how we see 'sex' itself which is more than just orgasms and genital play, it's so much more. During cancer treatments and other life-altering events, you might need to temporarily let go of traditional forms of touch/sex. We can become excited, aroused, release pleasure hormones in our body from so many different ways. There are erogenous zones all over our bodies such as our inner thighs, breasts, nipples, under the armpits, the neck, earlobes, feet and many more depending on your body. Orgasms, engorgement, ejaculation, becoming 'hard' or 'wet', these don't need to be your goal, but can also be experienced in more than one way. Pleasure, enjoyment, arousal, excitation and connection, that is where the fun can also be. Pleasure is pleasurable and our whole body can be pleasured!

Desire vs arousal

Desire (the wanting) I use interchangeably with libido. Desire/libido are the experience of *wanting* sex and pleasure. Desire has many words that can be used, such as lust, sex-drive, and essentially all refer to that *want* we have.

Arousal is the way our body responds when it's in pleasure, the changes in our body that show us we are in fact, enjoying and excited. Things like increased sensitivity, maybe we become wet, maybe we become hard, our heart rate increases, we breathe heavier and more.

Simply put, libido = wanting, and arousal = enjoying.

Treatments can affect our arousal as well as our libido, which I dive into in this book, but knowing the difference between these can be very helpful.

The magical word, intimacy

Disconnection from yourself and others is a common side-effect of cancer treatments for so many. You're not alone in this and here I introduce you to the magical word 'intimacy'. Imagine that you having sex or being intimate again with yourself, a date or a partner/s, is the goal or the prize. That prize is on the other side of a river, and to get to it, you need to build a bridge. How can you do that? Through intimacy, through touch and the other magical word *affection*.

I've heard many times from clients and people in my support group "we don't even touch each other anymore". Not only has sex gone, but so has the *intimacy*, and are we really going to want sex without that connection?

Intimacy and affection are small giants. Tiny little things that can mean the world, and build that bridge of connection. Things like hand-holding, a good-night kiss, a good morning hug, your arm around your partner in the kitchen, cuddling on the couch, touch for the sake of touch (not as a way to 'get somewhere'), massage swaps, maybe a cheeky butt-squeeze and grin, and the big one, WORDS OF LOVE.

When you want some touch or love? Here's a few ways to ask, without that pressure of it needing to lead to sex:

How to say it out loud.

- "Hey, I'd like to be closer to you, how about a cuddle?"
- "Can we snuggle together on the couch while watching this film?"
- "You up for some hand-holding while we walk to the shop?"
- "I'm loving you right now, thought I'd share."
- "You up for some underwear-on cuddling while we fall asleep? I miss connecting with you."
- "I'd love some touch/to touch your body, would you like a massage?"
- "I'm not wanting this to lead to sex, but some kisses and cuddles would be lovely if you're feeling like some connection?"
- "I'm checking you out right now, just wanted to share."

- "I'm running a bath to relax and wind-down from the day, would you like to join me for some down-time?"

Small giant steps towards that prize.

2. CONNECTION

When people hear the word 'connection', some assume it means something to do with sex. Well, that is not necessarily always the case as there are so many different types of meaningful connection in our lives, which I'll discuss here.

Connection could be the sharing of intimacy through affection with another, or with yourself. It can make you warm, bring you closer to someone, provide feelings of value and being loved. A hug from a friend, a hand-hold from a family member, even a simple smile from a stranger. Connection, belonging, it all can have a positive impact on us.

Why connecting is essential

I want to share a 'light bulb' moment I had during chemotherapy, one that helped me change a lot about the way I connected to those around me.

I was 4 months into chemotherapy and had just switched to having chemo weekly. It was a sweltering 38-degree Australian summer night and I walked out of a poetry reading with a friend, to go home. While walking, he hooked his arm through mine, as a sign of affection and connection. When his arm linked through mine, I noticed that I jumped at the touch. Noticing my reaction and how much I had been startled at the contact, it dawned on me. How long had it been since I had been touched in a way that was not medical, hurried and detached? Three weeks? Maybe four? I was so used to the non-intimate hands of nurses, oncologists, surgeons etc. who were not aggressive, but let's say, purposefully unaffectionate in their touch. It was a shock to receive this wonderful soft, intimate connection of an arm slipping through mine. I realised I had become an object of analysis and procedure, and was no longer one of affection. It was shocking to me and it also saddened me.

That was the moment I realised I was losing connection, that was the moment I saw I was becoming detached and I needed to be more vocal. The people around me were being respectful and careful not to touch me, due to how unwell I was. I loved everyone's respectful approach and care towards me as I was very, very sick. I'm grateful for their care, but I realised they also needed guidance from me, to know what was okay and when.

Realising the only touch I had been receiving was

medical, which I would switch off to and detach myself from, was one of those 'ahaaa' moments. I had realised how disconnected I'd become to my body and that I needed to make the first move and communicate. So, I beg you, educate those around you. Tell your friends they can hold your hand, your family members can put their arm around you, a partner or lover can snuggle with you on the couch. Be their guide for your connection. There are some examples on how to do that further on in this book.

3. LOSS OF SPONTANEITY

I honestly could not count the number of people I've heard mention that they wish they could go back to "the way it was", how they "want the spontaneity back".

Sure, while you're fighting cancer, you're not suddenly ripping each other's clothes off in the television commercial break. But it's not just cancer that can change our intimate patterns. This is also normal for people in longer term relationships and anyone experiencing any stressful life-event. Also, let's think about when you were having spontaneous sex, what was happening in your life? Was there more time with each other? More foreplay? More flirting? More affection? More intimacy? Less stress?

Spontaneous sex is not the only type of sex. Removing spontaneity gives way for intention. Sure, a little more planning might not get your juices flowing in an instant, but it shows love, thoughtfulness and caring. That's pretty hot! You can make planned sex and intimacy special, like an upcoming and exciting date. It gives you time to prepare, to make sure you're well rested and not hurried or rushed. This allows you to get in the right headspace, which will guarantee you a better time. Plus, planning can be a lot of fun and is totally psychological foreplay.

A sexuality educator I was listening to recently, discussing this topic brought up this question and it was another one of those 'ahaaa' moments with me. They asked "how many romantic movies show the caring, intentional long-term portions of relationships where couples spend their day 'doing life'. A film where they cook, do the dishes and crash in bed late at night exhausted after a full day's work?" I'm going to say, hardly any.

Romantic films usually show the first stages, meeting, dating, flirting, the new relationship energy, the excitement and adrenaline, and when you have time for so much fun. Life isn't always like that, but that doesn't mean you can't connect and have pleasure.

Sex can still be fun, pleasurable and connective, even if it needs a bit of planning.

4. COMMUNICATING'S HARD, BUT IMPORTANT

Please don't be down on yourself if you're struggling (whether you're a partner or the person diagnosed). Things are hard, things are different. It's okay, there are workarounds (which I'll get into soon). Ignore external pressures and expectations and focus on yourself and each other. Not only do our bodies and lives change from cancer, so do our roles. From partner to patient, lover to carer, friend to carer etc. You can get through it, together.

Silence is the enemy and can be common when we're finding things difficult. Fear and uncertainty are prevalent during treatments and we can withdraw from each other intentionally or unintentionally. It makes sense that we don't talk about the thing that's hard to talk about!

Fear of dating, meeting new people, of hurting a partner, not knowing how their/your new body works or not wanting to cause pain can all be reasons someone withdraws. Plus, your partner/loved one has seen you go through one of the hardest things of your life, be more unwell than ever, it's scary stuff.

For reasons above and more, not knowing how to

interact and pulling away is common.

For the people with the diagnosis, understanding what is happening in our body and communicating that? That can feel impossible. Either way, humans have not evolved to read minds, so you'll need to break the silence and share what's happening. So often, the concerns we have in our minds seem a lot bigger when they stay in our minds. Talking is key.

And while we're at it, please don't compare yourself to anyone else or any other relationships. It's the fastest way to unhappiness at any level and that includes comparing yourself to yourself, the 'pre-cancer you'. I call myself 'Tess BC' (BC = before cancer) when I'm in that loop. I often think of my pre-cancer body and mind, how I used to have less pain, more energy, body parts that used to be there, how I could remember things and focus on tasks, so you're not alone in this. I constantly remind myself, comparisons to others or the way things used to be won't change anything. It's such an easy pattern to fall into. I'm sorry to be so blunt as it's hard not to think about what has changed and how things used to be, but please try to think ahead. Cancer is different for everyone and every relationship is different.

There are millions of us fighting cancer, with suffering sexuality. It can be scary, but you don't have to do this alone.

Who to ask and how to ask

Communication with your loved ones isn't the only thing that's essential, but also communication with your treating team. Knowing who to ask about sexuality, positioning, care & *safety* is something most of us don't know.

<u>Here's a general summary.</u>

Gynaecologists work with people who have a vulva and/or vagina. Urologists work with those who have a penis. Gastroenterologists and colorectal surgeons work with the digestive system including bowel cancers. Haematologists work with blood and lymphatic cancers. You will also have medical professionals relative to your treatments such as a radiation oncologist for radiotherapy treatments, an endocrinologist for hormone treatments and the effects they have on our bodies and sexuality, and your oncologist who oversees your treatments. You will have a surgical team relative to the type of procedure you will be having. Psychiatrists are who to speak with regarding mental health and medications, including which medications have which impacts on your sexuality.

All of these people plus your nurses, your doctor or GP (general practitioner if you're in Australia) are all trained to answer your questions.

There are also people like me (OTs) who focus on sexuality, there's pelvic floor physiotherapists and OTs, there are sexologists and sex counsellors as well. You will need to ask; you will need to be your own advocate for your sexuality. But don't worry, if they're not sure how to best answer your question, they will find someone who is. Your care is their priority.

I hear you saying "sure Tess, it's easy to tell us to ask medical professionals questions, but *how* do you ask the questions?" The first step (asking) is the hardest.... But you can do it, I've got your back!

How to say it out loud.

- "What are the precautions I need to take regarding sexual activities during this treatment?"
- "Do I need to know about any sexual side effects from this treatment"
- "What do I and my partner/s need to know or do

regarding intimate activities?"

- "I'd like to ask a few questions about sex and intimacy during my treatment, in particular libido. Is there a more private space we could go to?"

- "Is there someone I can speak with, who can answer questions about sex during and after treatment?"

- "We/I would like to discuss intimacy during/after treatment. Can we organise a time? And with who?"

- "I'm experiencing some changes with my libido. Who is the best person to speak to?"

- "How will this treatment affect me/us intimately?"

- "I'm not sure how to ask this, but I have some questions of a more private nature, who can I speak with about that?"

- "Are there things I/we can do to help reduce any of the sexual side-effects from this treatment?"

If a healthcare professional isn't sure or cannot answer your question?

- "Thanks for letting me know, can you please ask someone who might be able to answer?"

- "Okay, can you please tell me who I can ask?"

Communicating with your partners

Pop-quiz, what am I?

We're not supposed to talk about it, you can't have too much of it, you can't have too little of it, it's used in nearly all marketing to sell but it's never presented accurately in the media, it's a part of human life, social media platforms shut you down for talking about it, people who are different, unwell, older, living with disability, are of different cultures and ethnicities are assumed to not have it or to want it, we receive no education on it yet we're supposed to magically be good at it and we're supposed to always want it....... Yup. That'd be sex.

You may feel from reading the above that you can't win, and sure, our culture doesn't exactly embrace open communication regarding sexuality, but reading this book is how you will learn.

In my experience as a sexuality educator (as well as from my own life), people who are able to talk between themselves about sex more openly, have much better sex. Why, you ask? Because communicating about how you're feeling and what you might enjoy, allows you to engage comfortably and pleasurably. It can also reduce feeling like you're forcing yourself, forcing someone else, or causing any possible harm. It's okay if things have changed, our bodies and pleasure always will. If we can learn how to communicate about what we do or don't want, things will be better. Remember, hand holding, eye contact, cuddles, snuggles on the couch, foot/body/hand massage, genital massage, oral genital play, assisting/giving masturbation, self-touch together, watching pornography together or reading erotic literature together, all of these things are sex and all of them are connective.

5. WHY LIBIDO DROPS

The two things I hear the most:

"I just don't want it anymore"
"It's like living with a friend"

I've been there and I am there. As I write this, the endocrine treatments I'm on have fizzled away the hormones that 'drive my drive' so to speak. It's tough, but it's not the end. Here I want to discuss how desire and intimacy work in the human body and the reasons we can experience drops in libido.

Here's the thing, desire/libido have a few layers to them. There's the physiological side, the psychological side and the neurological side. All of which can impact our libido.

The physiological side relates to the hormonal, physical and chemical changes in our body that treatments cause. That could be chemotherapy, medications, hormone treatments and others, which cause things like pain, dryness, changes in erection, fatigue and more. The psychological side relates to our emotions, patterns and stress. Both have an impact on our desire, and some are easier worked on than others.

The neurological side relates to how our brain is wired around what we do day to day, how we're feeling day to day/month to month, and influences how our brain is wired around things like libido. I discuss this more soon, but these three core aspects of ourselves (physiological, psychological & neurological) all impact our desire, the wanting.

It can be difficult to increase desire physiologically if we are still undergoing treatments such as hormone therapies, which impacts the way our body naturally works, like pushing a boulder up a hill. But that's not the end of it. If we're still on treatments and getting our 'drive' back to what it was isn't possible, there are still a few things that can be done to at least *improve* your desire (more on that later).

The psychological side is just as important, if not *more* important than the physiological. Did you know that stress impacts 100% of all human sexuality? 100%! A teeny tiny portion experience an increase in desire from stress, but most (I'm talking over 95% here) experience a drop in libido. And what's more stressful than cancer?

When we're stressed, we have less desire…when we have less desire, we're stressed. It's such a catch as the guilt and concerns about not wanting sex are contributors to us not wanting it.

But wait, there's more.

Our brain is our main sex organ. It's what's in between our ears, not our legs, that is our sex. And, as we all know, there are a lot of emotions and feelings that can occur in the back of our minds 24/7 and also play a large part in blocking our desire, 24/7.

Other than stress, another huge barrier to our wanting, is a sense of obligation or pressure that we *should* be wanting. I'll rephrase that. When we're tired, worried, stressed (even with a pre-cancer body), or forcing ourselves (I call it the 'should-brain'), our desire and libido drop, the 'wanting' just disappears. You're not going to want something that is an obligation. You're not going to want something that causes you emotional strain.

Just a few psychological barriers to your libido.
- Shame for not wanting sex.
- Stress or anxiety for experiencing changes in your sexuality.
- Guilt for asking a partner for sex.
- Guilt for saying no.
- Regret for saying yes.

- Awkwardness and distance as you don't want to 'hassle' your partner for affection.
- Stress & fear of living post diagnosis & recurrence.
- A sense of obligation and expectation that you should be sexual and having regular sex.
- Fear of hurting your partner.
- Financial and work stressors.
- Grief and loss for the way your body used to function.
- Feeling like you should be providing your partner with their needs (by the way, if your partner is desperate for sex, they can have sex with themselves, any time. Sex is never anything that is 'owed' to anyone).
- Feeling like you *should* be more sexual.
- Discomfort and stress as you don't know how to talk about things with your lover/partner.
- Anxiety/self-consciousness of your new body.

And so, so much more.

The core lesson I want you to understand from this, is that libido is extremely complicated and multi-layered. There is no quick magic-pill fix for our desire. I'm sorry if this is all doom and gloom right now, but I do have hope for you. Through understanding how our libido is affected on these levels, we can then work on rehabilitating it. And yes, you can (been there and done that), which I discuss in the next section in this book, and also guide people through libido recovery in my online course 'connection and cancer' (refer to the 'resources' section at the end of this book).

6. PLEASURE IS A BICEP (RECOVERING LIBIDO)

I'm Australian and I don't beat around the bush (Aussie slang for, I'm honest and to the point). I won't tip-toe around and fluff how hard this is. It's hard. I'm also here to give you hope.

Like a broken record, I mention that our brain is our largest sex organ and the best thing about it is that it's not solid concrete, forever stuck in its ways. I've worked in neurological rehabilitation in public and private hospitals working with brain injury, stroke, spinal cord injury and more, so I'm going to do my best not to get carried away in my neuro-speak. But here's a vitally important piece of knowledge for your future relationship and life overall.

Your brain can *change*. It's called 'neuroplasticity' and those of us who work in the neurosciences have a saying, "*Use it or lose it*". What this means is that the more we do something, the 'larger' the sections in our brain get which are dedicated to that area/to doing that thing. It's like the more you exercise your bicep, the larger and stronger it gets. The same thing happens with our neural pathways and the sections in our brain that are dedicated to doing the thing or feeling the thing. Here's the interesting part, the opposite also happens, the 'lose it' in that motto.

If we don't do something often, just like that bicep would get weaker without regular use, the pathways or connections in our brain get 'smaller' as they're getting used for other things (the things we are currently doing more often day to day). You're likely wondering why all of a sudden, you've stepped into neuro-speak, but hear me out as this is so important.

Our pleasure is a part of this process and so is our desire. Just like that bicep, we want to strengthen our pleasure pathways by *doing*! And this is where it all ties in.

Remember that bridge we want to build mentioned earlier? The small-giant steps towards the goal on the other side of the river? The wanting and having sex again? This is how we take that first gigantic and yet seemingly small step.

Focussing on *intimacy* as a way to neurologically 'rewire' our pleasure and wanting, is a way to achieve this. Cuddling, kissing, touching, words of love, all of these things I've been discussing throughout this book contribute to your feeling warm, safe and intimate with your partner/lover/yourself and can help reduce the pressure of it all. Plus, it's a way to start creating positive neural associations and remind your brain that you do indeed like and want touch.

I'll be sharing a few really fun, practical ways to do this shortly, but there's a little more explanation I want to give.

Without touch and connection, without affection and feelings of love, warmth and worth, why would we want sex?

Taking a step back, focussing on the little things can remove those psychological barriers to libido discussed earlier, to help you connect, communicate, and maybe then you'll start to feel less 'should-brain' and a bit more 'want-brain'. Differently said, removing the pressure of sex and re-introducing touch, intimacy and affection, is the start of the process that moves sex from something that we *should* do, to something we *want* to do.

Neurologically rewiring our desire, our libido, our pleasure, takes time and repetition of intimate touch, but it's also extremely simple and enjoyable.

Below I use partner-centric language, but want to confirm that if you're solo and wish to reconnect with yourself and your desire, the below strategies can also be followed with yourself individually, and are also applicable for persons in alternative relationship dynamics.

Where do we start?

Ignore the sex part for now, take it off the table for a timeframe (maybe a month or two), to focus on building that bridge and removing the psychological barriers to wanting. Don't worry, you're only banning sex with each other for a few months, you're welcome to have sex with yourself any time.

I'm sure I sound crazy, 'don't focus on sex to want the sex'. But our brains, our minds, our emotions and psychology are that first step. By removing sex all together from the equation, you're also removing that source of pressure, the 'should-brain', the grief, shame and anxiety. When we agree with a partner that we are temporarily taking sex off the table so we can reconnect, it frees up time for non-agenda'd touch. Touch and affection without the stress of it leading to sex, or going somewhere, allowing you to really enjoy the experience and is powerful for neurological change.

Organise with your lover, partner or yourself time for some touch preferably twice a week following the stages outlined below. This is called 'sensate focus' and is a technique used to reconnect people and increase desire going back to the 60's, created by researchers Masters and

Johnson. This process has incredible neurological benefits as it's slow and repeated. The perfect recipe for neurological change.

Stage 1: Start engaging in slow soft touch with each other (or yourself), but clothes on and all over the body. Avoiding typical erogenous zones such as breasts or genitals. But you're taking turns, so one of you is being touched and the other is doing the touch for a limited amount of time (maybe 10 mins each) and then you switch.

Stage 2: Next again is full body slow soft touch, starting with stage 1 touch (avoiding the typical erogenous zone initially). Then including the erogenous zones over clothing. Still taking turns in touching each other.

Stage 3: This is mutual touching; clothes are optional here. It's important you always start with the type of touch you were doing in stage 1, then 2, then 3 so our body and mind have time to relax and get into it. You're not going for the erogenous zones immediately and you want to avoid orgasms/climaxes and forms of penetration.

Stage 4: If everyone is feeling ready, proceeding through stages 1-3, this 4th stage involves nudity, full body contact and moving into positions that would look like how you would 'normally' have sex (without actually having it). After you've had a few 'sessions' of stage 4 and everyone is comfortable, moving onto having sex (whatever that looks like for you) with each other is fine.

If you keep these touch dates to a few times a week and for 20-40 minutes, you'll start to notice after a few weeks that you're actually looking forward to being touchy and intimate. I've done this myself after treatments to recover my desire and have personally guided others through this process, and it truly does have an effect. It's neuroscience.

The above 4 stages are a guide and depending on which therapist you see, can vary in what each stage entails and for how long you need to do them. For some the above may sound like something you can try. For others, reading is not doing, and even starting the process to have these conversations or integrate these strategies seems too hard. If that's you, please know I created an online program for couples called 'Connection & Cancer', where I guide and support people through each step of the entire process and more (refer to the 'resources' section). Doing is doing, and is where the change really happens, so I've got your back. In the course is a sensate program I designed specifically for people with cancer that spans over six weeks, and doesn't only rebuild desire, but also recovers pleasure sensation and body confidence. Six weeks is the sweet-spot for neurological change as it also allows time to go slow.

If the above doesn't seem achievable for you right now, focus on keeping your intimacy alive. Think of intimacy as the thing that keeps the coals burning, so re-lighting the fire is easier later on. Kiss for the sake of kissing, play the 2-minute game (described in the 'simple ideas for connecting' section), set a timer and slowly touch parts of each other's bodies. Relearn what you do and don't like. Explore, but also keep it simple. You want to remind your brain that touch and pleasure are things that you can enjoy. This is how we can recreate positive associations to touch and pleasure. We need to remind our brain that we are vessels of pleasure, that we enjoy touch. Giving ourselves time to understand how our new body works, and the above stages of touch offers slow and effective ways to do that.

There are plenty of affectionate partnerships out there who still struggle with low desire and libido. If this is you, the above sensate therapies are a great way to start that process of wanting again.

Medications + Herbs

I won't lie. A part of me didn't want to include the below information as, with everything, there are potential risks. However, it's important people know what's out there, and more importantly, learn about options while also learning that they might not be safe (or successful). When reading the below, know these are not direct clinical recommendations. Before trying any new medication or supplement you must discuss these options with your doctor and/or oncologist beforehand, to ensure your safety.

In the US, Vyleesi + Addyi are medications to offer support for people with hypoactive sexual desire disorder (HSDD). Although FDA approved, they have mixed results for people with low desire due to medications, treatments and illness, plus have quite a few potential side-effects. It could be worth looking into, but please talk to your doctor first as they may not be appropriate for you (or safe) to try. There are also natural herbs which are said to help things like desire and blood-flow, however it's important to know that some herbs can also influence hormone changes (like maca root, damiana, ashwagandha, L-arginine and fenugreek), so before considering anything you must chat with your doctor/oncologist first. *Especially* if you have a hormone receptive cancer, making sure to mention your treatment history and cancer type in these discussions.

When in doubt, the just described four-stage-libido rehab guide through sensate activities and neurological concepts is a safe (and effective) way to recover libido.

Anti-depressants

There are anti-depressants that lower libido, and are sadly the ones that are most often prescribed. It's unfortunately common, however, there are anti-depressants out there that don't have sexual side-effects. This is a conversation only to be had with your psychiatrist, and it's crucial for your wellbeing that these conversations are had with a trained mental health professional who knows you and your case. But please don't be afraid to ask if there are alternatives, because there are.

Your therapist needs guidance as to what's meaningful to you (love, intimacy, relationships, pleasure). A simple "what are my anti-depressant options that won't impact my sexuality or have sexual side-effects?", is all that is needed for the psychiatrist to make the right suggestions for you.

A shout-out to partners

Mismatched libido (when one person has a higher libido than the other) is tough. I support partners through so much shame, as they struggle with having more desire and libido while their partner is fighting cancer, and has less. There is a lot of guilt from this and people quite often do their best to hide their attraction to their partners and as mentioned, often looks like distance or disinterest. Libido isn't something that you can switch on and off at will. I know partners who hide when they masturbate from their partner, not wanting to expose them to anything uncomfortable, for feeling like a predator or being interpreted as putting pressure on their loved one. But self-pleasure doesn't have to be solo-pleasure. A partner can pleasure themselves with their loved one lying next to them, or even offering kisses or body touch. This can be beautiful and intimate. This can even influence greater connection and those lusty feelings.

People often simply want to be wanted and loved, and you can show love and affection without it having to lead to sex, which is what so many tools and strategies in this book offer.

Remember, you can have sex without having the sex!

7. REACTIVE AROUSAL VERSUS PROACTIVE AROUSAL

I've discussed mismatched libido, but I'd also like to discuss mismatched arousal. Remember, arousal is the way our body responds *in* pleasure, our enjoyment. Libido is the wanting and desire. As discussed earlier in this book, arousal responses could include things like an increase in heart rate, our pupils dilate, skin sensitivity increases, tissues become engorged, we become wet, we become hard and more.

Delayed arousal responses are extremely common from treatments and medications, and can also be caused by many psychological aspects like stress and nervousness. Just like we have the many layers (physiological, psychological and neurological) that can impact our libido, so do these layers potentially impact our arousal. What this can look like, is you don't 'want it as much' (or at all), it takes a lot longer for you to 'get into it' than it used to. That you notice it feels like maybe you're forcing yourself at the start, but after some time, things start to feel more enjoyable. Sound familiar?

I call this **'reactive** vs **proactive'** pleasure and arousal.

Reactive means, in *response* to something. You *react* to a thing or stimulus. With arousal and pleasure, that could look like only feeling aroused *after* you have been kissing and touching for some time. You're reacting to the touch and intimacy.

Proactive means something that happens *without* prompt or stimulus. It happens without needing something to react too. In pleasure and arousal this could look like you're watching television and all of a sudden, you're gagging for it. Or you walk down the street enjoying the sun on your face and you then notice your underwear is damp and the breeze feels soooo good!

Countless people feel their enjoyment of sex is gone forever, that they have lost their desire completely because their pleasure and arousal seem now absent (is no longer proactive). But in actual fact, it's just now reactive and it needs something to respond to and a bit of time to kick in. There's a gigantic difference between someone who doesn't enjoy sex at all versus someone who needs time to enjoy it.

I support many who think they cannot stand sex at all anymore and are desperate to reclaim this part of their life, and when I ask "So what do you do to warm-up before sex?" This question is followed by silence, a tumbleweed rolls past and that's the moment where I get my whiteboard out.

I'd like you (and anyone you're with) to grab a piece of paper and a pen, a notebook, or anything you can individually draw and write on. Now, draw a very basic XY graph (just a small graph is fine) with the Y axis labelled as 'arousal' and the X axis labelled as 'time'.

It should look something like this:

A
R
O
U
S
A
L

TIME

This graph is going to represent how much time we

need for our arousal and pleasure to kick-in, once we've started touching and playing either with ourselves or a partner. We're tracking our arousal response. As you move to the right, this indicates time passing. As you move upwards, this indicates your level of arousal increasing.

Imagine now, that you're getting sexy with yourself or a partner. This is where we're at the very start of the graph, where X & Y connect at the bottom left. I want you to draw a line on this graph, starting at this point, that shows what you feel your current arousal response is over time. You could get specific with this if you like, but mostly, let's just use this broadly as a guide and note that this graph could represent around an hour of time.

To repeat the task, imagine you're getting intimate with yourself or a partner. I want you to draw on the graph, a line representing what you think your arousal and pleasure response is like over time.

Here's an example of what this *could* look like:

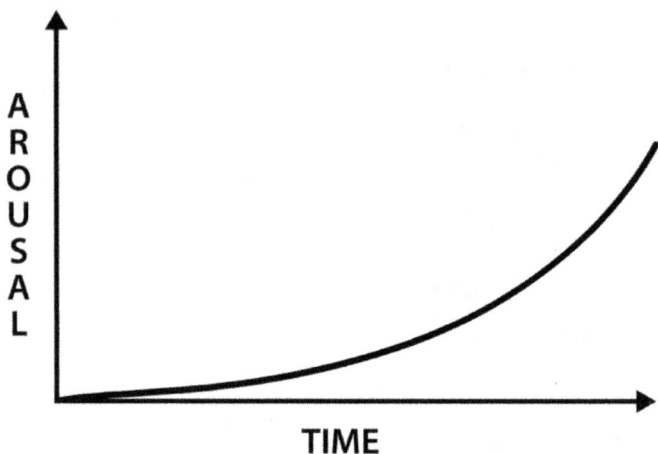

This graph shows that this person doesn't have an immediate arousal response (which is very normal during and after treatments), however after some time and a bit of lovin, they start to enjoy things more.

Now, if you're currently doing this with another person, I'd like for you to draw a second graph, and on this one, you're going to redraw your own line on it, and also in the same graph in another colour, copy this other person's line into it also. Then, circle where those lines intersect (if they do). So, you have two (or maybe more if you're with multiple people) lines on the one graph, giving us a comparison.

It *could* look something like this:

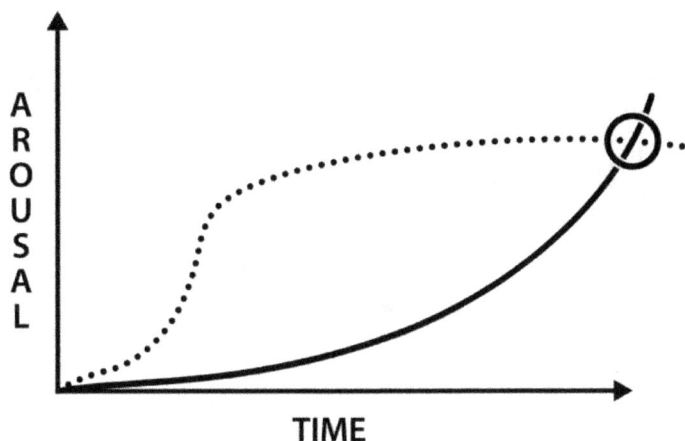

TIME

For many people the lines vary quite a bit and for others, not so much. There's no right or wrong here, we're simply visualising the invisible processes within our body. No matter how similar or different these lines are, it's extremely rare that the lines would be identical.

Why? Because we are all different, as is our sex and our pleasure. But the two parts of this graph I want you to focus on is the part where the lines intersect, and the space in between the lines which I've highlighted on the next graph.

The space in between the lines represents the time in your connection and intimacy, where you're mismatched in your pleasure and arousal. One of you is more aroused, faster. What we want to do is get you to the point where those lines intersect, because this is your happy spot. This is where sex is pleasurable and enjoyable for all involved. This is the sexy goldilocks zone.

That highlighted space is the guide for you to know how much more time and attention one person needs, so you can get to that intersection point for mutual enjoyment. This is fantastic to know, because guess what? If you need more time and attention, we can give you more time and attention!

Brainstorm together, right now, some things you can do together or alone, that will help the person who needs a little more time, to feel relaxed, feel calm and feel sexy. What things could you do at the start of your play and intimacy that will help this person arrive into their body and pleasure, so you're both on the same page? Is it a massage? A warm bath followed by some soft touch? Is it soft kisses on the neck and lower back? Is it watching some porn together? Use that space in the graph, the mismatch in your pleasure as a guide on how to get your pleasure to match. This is how sex becomes more enjoyable for everyone and ties into the thing that will contribute you to wanting it more. Remember that bicep? The wanting? If we're having lovely experiences with ourselves/partners, we will be creating those positive pleasure neurological associations and want it more!

For people doing this individually, look at the curvature of your line/arousal. Is there a lot of time where you aren't feeling pleasure and those arousal responses? Think about your self-pleasure practices. Are they rushed? Do you go straight to the genitals? Do you feel frustration that you're not 'getting there' fast enough or at all? Brainstorm for yourself, are there things you could do to help you drop into your body and its pleasure before your self-pleasure? Erotic dancing, full body touch, porn, erotic literature, what can you integrate into your pleasure practices so you can really connect with your pleasure and arousal?

The next time you're planning a sexy date with yourself or another, remember the graph, your reactive arousal and look at these things you've brainstormed. Plan a few of these at the start of your connection, to give the person who needs a little more time and attention just that. This is how we all have a better experience, this is how we can ensure a pleasurable experience for all, even with a slower arousal response.

This can be tricky for some people, and the idea of receiving more attention than the other may be surprisingly difficult. We're raised in a culture to believe that sex is some form of an exchange. Well, it's not. You don't give, *just* so you can receive. There should be no agenda in sex. If you need to receive more attention, more touch and more focus in sex, please know you're not a selfish lover. You don't need to 'return the favour'. Sex is a gift and doesn't need to be strictly two-way all the time. Remove the agenda, so you can access your pleasure.

If you drew a comparison graph and the multiple lines on it don't intersect, perhaps one of your lines looks almost horizontal, that's okay. That happens and you're definitely not the only one. Please know there is hope. You can rehabilitate your arousal and work towards getting those lines to intersect, towards getting your line to move upwards quicker. How? By doing those sensate activities detailed in the 'pleasure is a bicep' section or my online libido recovery masterclass 'connection and cancer (detailed in the 'resources' section). It's all about neurologically rewiring our pleasure pathways, and through those sensate techniques and other strategies in this book, you can.

Some people may experience numbness or desensitisation on their vulva. Consider having a chat to your doctor about trying a 'scream cream' which is a prescription cream locally put onto the clitoral and vulva area 30 minutes before intimacy. It helps get blood-flow to the area and enhance sensitivity (blood is everything!), which can help influence delayed arousal responses. If you are someone with genital herpes, let your doctor/pharmacist know so they can make up a special formula, as for some people, the standard creams can cause breakouts.

If you love the idea of intimately playing with each other, touching and reconnecting, but aren't sure how, I share a list of ideas shortly in the upcoming section 'simple ideas for connecting'. In particular, 'chatty massage', the '2-minute game' and 'active receiving' are worth considering.

A quick note on exercise.

A study which was done comparing the impacts of light to moderate exercise in increasing sexual satisfaction, had two groups. One where people had to go for a quick jog before having a sexual experience and then rating it, versus people that didn't exercise and rated their sexual experience (the sexual experience was everyone watching the same erotic film). Most of the people that went for a jog beforehand had a much greater satisfaction score compared to those that didn't. It wasn't a huge study, but worth mentioning as the results make perfect sense. Exercise gets blood-flow to your pelvis and deeper genital structures, increasing sensitivity, pleasure and tissue engorgement, all the things that make up arousal! If you're able to time your sexy-time after you have some exercise, it may genuinely help quicken and intensify your arousal response time.

Please do not read this as me saying all you need to do is go for a jog and your sex will be perfect. Exercise is something that can help, but is not a cure. It is still important you sit down with yourself and/or your partner and do the above arousal graph and brainstorm together. Going for a brisk walk before touching and getting intimate so you're/you're both on the same page could be the difference between having a good time, and a great time.

8. HOW TREATMENTS AFFECT YOUR SEX LIFE

I thought I'd share a little about my experiences during treatments, to give a little context as to how sexuality can be affected.

Chemotherapy gave me labia ulcers and vaginal pain which made even a fingertip of penetration cause unbearable pain. Haemorrhoids prevented anal play and nausea had me wanting to keep still while constantly sipping on frozen cokes for instant relief. Mouth ulcers and bleeding gums had tasks such as eating challenging, so kissing was definitely not on the table. Endocrine treatments gave me low libido and vulvovaginal atrophy so bad, there were days and weeks I was unable to walk, sit-down, or wear underwear or pants (I haven't ridden my bicycle in years). I also have joint and bone pain and regular migraines. Chronic pain from radiotherapy and fatigue, drain tubes, surgery sites, and so much more. As you can imagine during these times, sexual activities were not something I was craving. However, with the guidance in this book (and in particular the next section), you will find some solutions and ideas on how to be intimate when perhaps you're not wanting typical forms of sex.

It's important to note that it's not just treatments which can lower our libido, cause changes in arousal and orgasm, but also medications. It's okay, you may still be able to enjoy a lot of pleasure, maybe even have orgasms (just different ones) in ways that might surprise you. Also, this is an important time to remember, you can still have pleasure and arousal without having to reach climax. Again, I repeat, pleasure is pleasurable!

One of the most common lessons I teach and other sexuality therapists teach, is that sex is more than your genitals, sex is more than your orgasm. Sex is your body, your connection, your arousal, your pleasure, your touch, your giving and your receiving.

9. SIMPLE IDEAS FOR CONNECTING

I keep saying connection is possible, even with the changes in our body and low libido but *how* is connection possible? Below I've listed and described some activities that I've taught, read about and love to do - and are my top picks for you to try yourself. It's not an exhaustive list, but will give you a start (i.e., trust yourself and you can decide what works for you). Not all will appeal to you, that is fine. They are varied enough so that hopefully there's something for everyone that seems appropriate to try. These are a lot of fun on a date-day, to explore, connect, have pleasure, affection and fun (and still have pleasure and sexyness), even if your 'normal' form of having sex isn't something you're wanting right now. Most importantly to know, is that even if you're not having and wanting sex right now, staying connected and affectionate with yourself and your partner is one of the best ways to ensure you'll get it back!

These activities can be done to the level that is right for you, with the person that is right for you. These can be done with a close friend, your carer, by yourself, partners and even family members! It's time to *really* connect. Here's a few ways to do this.

Q&A

I am obsessed with this verbal game and full credit to Roger Butler from Curious Creatures who created it. It's so useful and fun to play if you're in a position where you want to communicate with someone, but it's hard to bring up an awkward topic or start a conversation. It's also great to play any time anywhere, and I love it in social or private settings. It's so simple yet an incredible way to deeply communicate and connect with strangers, loved ones, friends and everyone else. Remember, your brain is your largest sex organ and the psychological barriers to our libido can be one of the main barriers. This game is a godsend for us feeling emotionally connected and safe, and these are the drivers for our sex-drive! During many of my treatments, I struggled (and still do) to keep up with conversations that involved more than two people as the brain-fog/cancer-brain had my attention span so low. I also struggled at times to have conversations about how I was feeling and where I was at. I often played Q&A as a way to be able to listen to one person at a time, and still have valuable, connective conversations with the people around me. I also play it one-on-one to have meaningful conversations with a partner or friend, while communicating was/is so difficult. Simply put, Q&A makes good conversation great, and when you're struggling, it's a life-saver.

How it works.

Someone asks a question, any question, such as: How was your day? How are you feeling in your body? What do you love about your partner right now? What is your relationship to your sex? Do you like cake more than ice-cream? Anything.

The person sitting to the left of the person who asked the question, answers it first. When they are finished, it goes to the next person to the left, finishing with the person that asked it. If you're in pairs, the person who asked the question, answers it last.

There are a few extra rules:
- Every answer is perfect.
- Every question is perfect.
- No interrupting someone's answer, wait until they have told you they are finished answering, before sharing your thoughts.
- You can 'pass' on a question (or make something

up!).

- You can call 'Tangent' or 'Time' by making a 'T' symbol with your hands. This indicates that someone may be off on a tangent or taking too much time to answer. We always say "thank you" for a 'T'.

- The person who asks the question, always answers it last.

It may seem strange, having a verbal Q&A game in a book about connection and the importance of intimacy, but there's a theme here. Cancer interrupts life, which includes relationships. Medications, fatigue, nausea, stress, it all interferes and open communication for some can seem too hard. Try this game, try it a few times, it was and still is, a 'go-to' for me, when I want to connect.

Where? You can play it anywhere. Try it in the bath, the couch, at dinner, in the car, a BBQ, your fortnightly or monthly relationship check-in, or a few rounds at the end of the week to see how you're going. It's a beautiful time to be honest, because the rules are that you can't be interrupted and every answer is perfect.

This is also your saving grace if conversations are hard,

paying attention is tricky and keeping up with multiple people talking at once. If you let people know what you need and where you're at, they will most likely help you out. I noticed social chatter was a way for people to let me know that 'everything was fine'. But it wasn't, I couldn't concentrate, I couldn't follow the conversation, I quickly forgot what people were saying and I got super stressed. As soon as I mentioned I needed conversation to slow down, that's exactly what happened. Remember, you will need to let people know what you need, and they will be grateful for the guidance. Q&A is a brilliant way to have social structure, and still offer wonderful connections with everyone present.

Little, lovely treats

Sit down and write a list of 5 - 10 things that are small and easy to do, that make you feel special or connected to yourself. Little, lovely treats. If you have a close friend or loved one, get them to do the same, write a list of little lovely things they enjoy. This could be a foot massage, a bath, a favourite wine, a nice cheese with salami and a childhood film (my personal favourite), moisturising each other's hands/backs/necks/chests, looking at photos together, a blindfolded touch experience, a game of loving Q&A (just described in this section) or dancing to your favourite music.

So, when a time comes, when you're feeling like you would like to connect, be intimate, share affection and don't know what to do? Get the list out and see what you're/you're all in the mood for.

All of these small treats should ideally be things that can be done in your home or very close to where you're staying, and don't take a lot of energy. You want your energy to be spent on connecting and enjoying yourself and others' company, not setting up or travelling to a location.

These 'small treats' lists are your go-to. When you're stuck in your head or having a bad day, get the list out. Soak your feet and moisturise them, do yoga, have a self-pleasure session or pleasure a partner, eat an entire pizza when those taste-buds are back online or get your favourite film and a pot of your favourite tea. The point is that you want an easy way to feel special involving yourself, and possibly those close to you. Simple, sensual, special treats that connect you with yourself/others.

Warming and calming

This small yet intimate task can really let you relax, unwind and get connected. A gentle, beautiful way to connect with yourself or with someone else, is by enjoying a warm bath. Relaxing in a body of warm water (not too hot!) has so many positive effects on the body. Muscles relax, our nervous system down-regulates (relaxes), it can reduce stress, muscle tension eases, pain can lessen, blood circulation improves, the list goes on. Add a cup of tea, a glass of wine, something playing on a screen you can see or some quality Q&A (see earlier in this section) if you have a 'bath-buddy' with you.

The waterless bath

Baths not your thing or you don't have one? I have for you, the waterless bath experience. Pop your electric blanket on a nice low setting or warm up a heat pack on the couch and create a warm snuggly cocoon for yourself or for you and your pet, child, friend or lover. The intent is to create warmth, intimacy, safety and connection - baths are not essential for this, but feeling safe and snuggly is.

A royal bathing

Credit for this idea goes to my primary carer, who 'softens' the daily activities to connect and show love, and has also used this technique when caring for a friend while undergoing treatments for brain cancer (spoiler, they loved it!). Is your partner, lover, friend or carer helping you with your personal care? Such as dressing, washing or even simply helping you dry your feet after the shower? If this is the case, every once in a while, ask the person assisting with your care to take their time with it. Turn it into an almost worshipping, lovingly sensual dressing or bathing. Imagine the treatment someone might get in a luxury ancient Roman spa.

Slowly wash the feet, slowly caress and wash the back, take your time enjoying putting clothing on someone, let the materials softly brush over the skin. Attention and intention are drivers of pleasure and going slowly allows this to happen. Yes, we are often time poor and we go into 'automatic mode', however this is a lovely five-minute task which can be added into daily life quite easily and shows care, love and affection. This small activity acts as a reminder to each other, you're not in a clinical environment, you're not a nurse going through the rounds with a patient, you're caring for someone, someone you care about. Be soft, be gentle, be present. What a treat and what a connector. And it only needs to take an extra five minutes or so.

A simple good night kiss

Life is hectic and a cancer diagnosis doesn't lighten the load. Finances, appointments, family life, medications, symptoms and more, can fill up the days. The only time you may actually see a partner or lover is at the end of the day. If this is you, think about taking five minutes, when you're in bed together getting ready for sleep. Lie down facing each other and look into each other's eyes. Touch noses if you like, hold hands, intertwine feet, hold eye contact, share a good-night statement, breathe together or share a kiss on the lips. It's a time where you're both settling down and both in the same spot, it's a great time to use it to connect.

Don't go to bed at the same time as the person you live/share space with? That's okay, ask that you get 'tucked-in' or tuck your partner in. Get the blankets up to their chin, wish them good night, give them a kiss and a few words of love. It's just such a sweet thing. And if you don't share a house with your loved ones? Sweet, loving good night text messages mean the world!

Self-pleasure

Our entire bodies are capable of pleasure and giving yourself some time, some touch and love is a beautiful way to connect with yourself and get those happy chemicals flowing. During treatments you may be tired, stressed, sore, in pain or feeling flat. Whether you're single or partnered, a lovely way to calm and connect with yourself is to give your body, soft, loving touch. This can, but doesn't necessarily need to involve your genitals or you getting aroused. Our bodies are complicated things and treatments can make our body almost feel like a stranger, so getting to know it again can be wonderful.

Give yourself some time, show yourself you're special and set yourself a date. Be it once a fortnight, once a week, or whenever you feel slightly motivated. It's nice, the first few times if you try to leave genitals out of it, just to see what it's like to focus on your body in a different way. We don't give ourselves enough one-on-one time and this is most definitely the case for personal intimate touch. Be curious, explore, hug yourself, scratch, tap, softly touch the skin, find what your body is and isn't enjoying, what it does and doesn't enjoy at that moment. I'm a firm believer that offering ourselves self-pleasure and understanding our bodies is essential for us to be able to connect with others. Regardless if you're partnered or not, having some time with yourself is healthy, it's calming, and it's connecting.

Massage swaps

This may seem like a strange thing to recommend in regards to intimacy and pleasure, but hear me out. Touch, care, love and affection are all things many of us forget about during and after treatments. If you're unsure of what your body wants in an arousal, erotic sense, your immediate fallback plan can be massage. Having someone massage you, gives focus on physical, attentive touch without that pressure of it needing to lead to sex. It's pleasurable, it's intimate and gets you connected (and it feels so good!). Massage swaps can also act as an 'ice-breaker', if you're with a partner or on a date and it's been a while since you've touched each other (which is common). This is a lovely and accessible way to ease back into a physical and touch based dynamic without the pressure to 'perform' or 'be sexy'. If you're not partnered and want some touch, but aren't sure how? There are many very skilled professional massage therapists out there, even the 'pop-in' 10-minute massage parlours have amazing touch and anything that connects you to your body and feels good, is a win.

Another amazing benefit of doing massage swaps, is it's a way for a partner or lover to get used to touching your changed body. So often, I support partners through their fear and anxiety of hurting their partner by touching them. A simple massage can be a way to have your partner touch your body and even start to explore areas they are hesitant to touch (like surgery sites or scars). With a little encouragement, direction and permission from you, these fears and anxieties can be overcome, together.

An undressing ritual

How we see ourselves and also, the fear of being naked in front of another person (and ourselves) can greatly impact our intimacy and also, libido. Undressing rituals are a method of removing clothing for yourself, or another, in a way that is gentle while allowing space for nervousness and shyness, while inviting acceptance and positive regard. You can do this solo by yourself in front of a mirror as a way to get used to your new body, or with a date or partners.

How it works.

There's a lot of scope for variety here so feel free to bend and change this to suit you, but here's the basics. Standing in front of a mirror or someone else, you choose one item of clothing at a time to take off, and as you remove it you make a personal statement. Something that is true, that is how you feel, but also as a way to process, release and move towards acceptance. It's a neat psychological trick and can be wonderful. If you're doing this with a partner, take turns, so after you remove an item of clothing and make a statement, they do the same. Then it's your turn again, and so on.

By statements I mean things like;

- As I remove my shoe, I let go of how hard I am on myself.
- As I take off my shirt, I let go of my self-consciousness.
- Removing my belt is me removing the restrictions of society's ridiculous beauty standards.
- As I remove my bra, I welcome in love and acceptance of my body.
- As I take off my scarf, I release my fear.

- By taking off my pants, I am freeing myself of anxiety.
- By removing my pink sparkly cowboy hat, I am letting go of my tiring day.

Or, if that form of statement doesn't feel right, you could try positive words as you remove clothing and show parts of your body:

- As I look at my arm, I notice the smooth skin I have.
- While looking into the mirror, I'm loving the freckles I have on my face.
- With my chest exposed I feel an appreciation for being alive.
- As I look at my genitals, I notice the awesome curls in my pubic hair.
- As I see my stomach, I see scars/marks of me living, and making it through.
- While looking at my lower back, I like the curve where it joins my bottom.

I have done this by myself in front of a mirror, with a long-term partner and also on a date. It was surprisingly effective on the date, as I was very self-conscious about my body and didn't know how to transition from clothed to well, not-clothed. We both took turns slowly removing an item of clothing, we looked into each-other's eyes, we were honest and it was magic. It helped me relax and it helped them understand how I was feeling and how I was struggling.

Go slow. If you're doing this alone in front of the mirror, it can be quite confronting. Don't feel like you need to fully undress, you may need to do this gradually over time. You could remove one additional item of clothing in the mirror to look at and love each time you do this, so it's nice and slow. I've done it several times alone, as a way to slowly look at myself and get used to my changed and abnormal body. I cried a lot, but it truly helped me with body acceptance and processing my grief for the body I used to have. Follow yourself, breathe and trust that you can stop if you need to. If you're with someone and you don't want to get naked, you can remove 'imaginary' items of clothing (like an orange feather boa, a sequin vest, rainbow suspenders etc.) or simply ask to stop. You could also do this with someone, where you take turns in removing an item of clothing off of the other person, while making positive statements about their body. Or maybe you choose the item of clothing on yourself to remove and your partner/date shares statements of love and appreciation of that particular body part. The best part of this activity is that there's room to change this to what feels right for you, at the pace that's right for you.

Chatty-massage

If you're liking the ideas in this book about communicating more about what you want and giving more feedback in intimacy and pleasure, but aren't really sure how to do that, this one's for you. 'Chatty massage' is very simple, and is the perfect way to get better at figuring out what you want or don't want, and also, how to ask for it. Plus, this is another excellent activity to do, if your partner is feeling a little hesitant to touch your body, because they're scared of hurting you.

How it works.

Easiest done in pairs, one of you is the 'masseuse', and the other receives the 'massage'. But there's a twist. The person lying down, the one receiving the 'massage' is actually directing the masseuse on what to do. Sounds easy right? Well, there's a little more to it.

The person who is receiving direction, the 'masseuse'

is only able to do exactly that, receive and follow directions. They cannot take over the experience or offer what they *think* the person receiving might enjoy. They can only follow the directions given by the person lying down who is 'receiving' the massage. The most important part of this however, is that if the masseuse/person following directions doesn't hear something along the lines of "keep going" or "I like this, continue please" or a new instruction, they must stop touching the person giving the directions all together by gently removing their hands and waiting (in silence) to receive the next instruction.

Why does the person have to stop touching after 10 seconds of silence you ask? For the person who is receiving the directions, this is a lesson in being guided in touch, in taking feedback and more importantly, not making assumptions as to what the other person may want and 'winging it'. For the person receiving the massage/giving directions, it allows them to learn how to ask for what they'd like and how to communicate if they'd like something to stop, continue or to change. It's powerful stuff. It's also an incredible way for them to really explore their body and to learn what they do and don't like at the pace that's right for them.

Giving feedback and knowing how to receive it during intimacy is the thing that makes a good time, a great time. But we're not taught how to talk about sex or our bodies. We're definitely not taught how to explore our likes and dislikes in a safe and compassionate way. The world would be better if we were. Chatty massage (as simple as it seems) is your way to flex those communication muscles and learn so much about your and your partner's pleasure.

If you're not sure where to start, try doing it together sitting on the couch and just on the hand or shoulders to start with. Or have a clothes-on play together while you get used to how it works. You could even set a timer so you have 5 or 10 minutes each of giving and receiving while you're trying it out. You can start by exploring things like soft touch on your arms, maybe scratchy touch on your back, massage touch on your neck and thighs. Soft kisses on your lower back. Feel free to get creative as the person following directions is going to stop if you don't ask for it to keep going, or ask for something to change. This is the safety mechanism, so you both can feel free to relax and have a bit of fun with it.

You may be thinking that the more difficult role in this is the person who's lying down and giving the directions.

Funnily enough, when I work with partners together and I teach them this activity it's the complete opposite. It's the person receiving directions and having to stop and withdraw touch after 10 seconds of silence that struggles the most! Due to this, I'm going to repeat the rule as it's surprisingly tough for people, but is so important. If the 'masseuse' doesn't hear a direction after 10 seconds, they must stop what they're doing, remove their hands and wait. This is what will help the person giving direction do exactly that, as they will *have* to give you direction when you stop. So much of our intimacy is guess-work and with the impacts of cancer treatments, clarity and communication could never be more important. Stopping the touch after a short amount of time is a way to help each other practice giving and receiving feedback and most importantly, tuning in to what you do and don't want at the time.

It will 100% feel clunky and awkward at first, just like everything else we try in life for the first time. Don't worry too much about it as this is play, and yes play can be clunky, but it can also be fun. Have a laugh and have another go. Communication is the number one sex move, and this activity is the perfect way to practise.

The two-minute game

Finally, we learn about the two-minute game! Life coach Harry Faddis created the 'three-minute game' and I was taught the 'two-minute game' from Roger Butler at Curious Creatures, and it's simply brilliant. This game is suitable for those experiencing treatment and their loved ones, is great when you have no idea how to connect with someone or where to start and is a wonderful way to gently get to know each other's bodies again.

Here's the rules.

- Set a timer or an alarm on your phone for two minutes.
- Pick who goes first, then that person asks for something they would like for 2 minutes (some examples are listed shortly).
- If you all agree, start the timer and give the person whatever they asked for.
- When the timer goes off, completely stop what you're doing.
- Then it's the next person's turn to ask for something they would like for two minutes.
- If everyone agrees, start the timer and go.

- Once the timer goes off, again, stop what you're doing.
- And repeat.

That's it. Really, that is the game. So simple, yet so effective. You can play it for as long as you like - 10 minutes or an hour, or however long you have energy and are having fun. Time can really fly when playing this game.

Also, this game can be played with anyone, not just someone you're in a relationship with. It could be a friend, family member, carer and doesn't have to be in pairs. There are so many ways to connect, to touch and be touched, which this game can help you discover.

One of the first (out of possibly hundreds) times I played this, I wasn't sure what to ask for. So, of course, I asked for a shoulder massage. Then, that became a slow back scratch. Then full body soft touch and I was amazed at how starting simply and being left wanting more (thanks to that timer) guided me to what I would like next. Asking for what you want can be difficult at first, but this game allows you to develop that skill with practice. Asking for what we want is such an essential skill to have during cancer treatments (and always).

A common question when introducing the two-minute

game in workshops is, "what happens if someone asks for something you don't want to do?" Say "no-thank you" with a smile and discuss an alternative (such as touching the chest or back rather than genitals). It's okay. Wait, it's more than okay, it's wonderful to say 'no'. Saying what we don't want is equally (maybe more) important than saying what we do want. The goal is to find that optimal place where everyone is happy giving and receiving.

Here's a few reasons why this game can work for you:
Our genitals aren't always up for being played with, so when it's your two minutes, ask for something that doesn't include them (you have your whole body).

This game can allow connection, even with different levels of libido. Someone might want sexual touch for two minutes and if you're happy to give it, great! Your two minutes could be something that suits your mood such as "tell me your favourite joke using your hand as a puppet". The possibilities are endless and you can ask for exactly what you want, while easily avoiding what you don't want.

Bodies impacted by treatment can change dramatically and unpredictably, be it sensation, arousal, pain, surgical sites etc. This game allows you to relearn how your body works or doesn't work (where those desensitised parts are, where it's sore, where it's pleasurable, how toys or lubes feel).

If you're playing this with a partner and are worried about where things may lead to? Take 'typical' sex off the table for the entire game. You could have a 'no genital contact' rule or even leave your clothes on. Remove the pressure to perform or get aroused. Obligation & expectation are the enemy of arousal, feeling safe and relaxed is its catalyst. Get creative, enjoy yourselves without that pressure. You can enjoy pleasure from soft intimate touch anywhere on the body.

The two-minute game has many communication benefits and can act as a gentle ice breaker. With changed sexuality and changed intimacy (with or without illness), can come distance and avoidance. Talking about sex is not easy, especially when things are different. This game gently offers a way to help navigate those tricky feelings while also acknowledging the elephant in the room. While we're at it, let's erase any feelings of 'being selfish' or 'a taker'. Asking for your neck to be gently kissed for two minutes, or to be told why this person loves you for two minutes, is simply playing the game. It can seem difficult, but remember, you have to ask, it's the rules! Through my work as a sexuality and consent workshop facilitator, I'm always shocked at how many people tell me that they have never asked for what they want before. Practice makes perfect and it does get easier the more you do it.

Here's a list of things you could ask for, for your two minutes:

- Can you please lower the lights, put some relaxing music on that I would like, bring me water and join me on the couch in two minutes?
- Hold my hand and tell me how you're doing for two minutes.
- Massage my (insert body part here) for two minutes.
- Starting at my neck, ever so softly touch my entire body, back to feet over two minutes.
- Tell me about your day through interpretive dance.
- Put on a song and show me your silliest/favourite dance move.
- Make me a cup of tea in two minutes.
- I would like to cuddle for two minutes.
- I would like to offer you a shoulder massage for

two minutes (that's still your two minutes, but if you're not up for being touched, you can touch others. It's all about what YOU want).

- Massage my head.
- I would like to stroke your hair with your head in my lap.
- Lightly touch my beautiful bald head for 2 minutes.
- Gently kiss my neck/chest/thighs/back for two minutes.
- Show me how you like to be kissed, for two minutes.
- Kiss my face and tell me things you love about me for two minutes.
- Softly breathe on my entire body, ending with my genitals for two minutes (YUM!).

If you're thinking, "ugh, whatever Tess. Some of us don't know how to just simply know what you want and ask for it." You're right, I hear you. None of us are taught this, but I have a solution for you. A beautiful baby-step towards the 2-minute game and flexing those 'asking' muscles, is by playing the previous activity 'chatty massage'.

Active receiving

'Active receiving' is a way to connect with a lover/partner to the level that is right for you, when you're not feeling sexy or like having sex, and maybe need a little bit more time to get those feelings flowing.

It's a one-way touch experience, and a great way to enjoy touch. I'll explain a little more. There are many expectations and misconceptions in intimate activities, and a super common one is that it should always be a two-way experience. You give and receive pleasure at the same time. Well, this doesn't necessarily always have to be the case, and I offer you a wonderful way to connect in a one-way touch format, very similar to 'chatty massage' mentioned previously. This is wonderful for people with mismatched libido, delayed arousal responses (detailed in the 'reactive versus proactive arousal' section), if someone is not wanting to receive intimate touch or may not know what they want at that moment, but would love to see a partner have pleasure and enjoy themselves.

How it works.

Someone lies/sits down (or is in any comfortable position), asks for what type of touch they want, and constantly directs that person in how they touch them. The other person does exactly what they are being told to do. That's it! It's incredibly fun and accessible.

Imagine the person giving the touch and receiving the directions has no mind of their own, they are an inanimate object that only responds to commands. For the person following instructions, it can free you from that common brain chatter ("am I doing this right? Are they enjoying this? Are they pretending?"), as you're just doing what you're told.

Some examples of directions the person who is receiving touch (and giving all directions) could give are: "Massage my shoulders. Can you now scratch my back? Yum, thanks, can you go slower and a bit firmer? Softly touch my body up and down, neck to feet with your fingertips and don't stop until I say. Now, lightly pinch my inner thighs. Breathe cool breath on my nipples." Anything you want, just ask.

Unlike in chatty massage where the person following directions stops all together if they don't hear anything after a short while, in 'Active Receiving', the person giving the touch can check in to see if it's how the receiver wants it ("How is this pressure? Would you like me to move my hands faster or slower?") *without* stopping. The person following directions doesn't change anything, doesn't alter any style without being directed. If the person giving touch doesn't receive any directions for a while and isn't sure if this is still what the person receiving still wants? Keep doing what you were last asked to do and ask the question "how could you enjoy this more?"

Similar to chatty massage, this is an incredible skill to learn in the bedroom. Giving directions, asking for what we want, checking in with a lover to get feedback on their level of enjoyment, communicating your desires, all of this leads to better communication and better sex. If you get tired? Simply stop the activity whenever one of you wants. The goal is to enjoy receiving and to enjoy giving. 1 minute, 10 minutes, 20 minutes, it's all perfect.

If you're unsure, give it a go, clothes on, on the couch, using just an arm or hand. Practice following directions, practice giving directions, practice checking in and identifying what you want. There is no goal here, just to have a touch experience, to give or receive pleasure, and enjoy connecting with a partner. It may feel clunky at first, but with practice it flows very easily and you will be amazed at how much you learn about your partner and their body (and yours!).

If this sounds like fun to you, but asking for what you want and giving directions seems a bit daunting, or taking directions and not being the one driving the experience sounds tough, I recommend playing 'chatty massage' or the '2-minute game' a few times first, before jumping into this activity. I say this only because it won't be enjoyable if you're still getting used to these styles of intimate communication. Those two activities are a wonderful (and fun!) way to develop these amazing sexy skills.

10. TIPS FOR LOVED ONES

Seeing a loved one go through cancer is tough, and so can knowing what to say or how to act. Whether you're a carer, friend, family member or partner, there are ways to offer connection without overstepping a line. And don't worry, we won't break!

Yes, caution is (very) necessary and the medical team must tell you about all of the risks involved in all treatments. People undergoing chemo, surgeries, radiotherapy, we can be seen as easily hurt, fragile or dangerous, and rightly so. There are many side-effects of treatments, some of them are mental and some of them are physical. However, let's remember this: connection is always important, and even if someone's body and mind are changing, there are still ways to be there with someone.

It can understandably be hard to know what to do. It's also normal, when seeing a loved one be so unwell, to want to avoid causing any other harm and through that, create physical distance. That might look like reducing touch and physical contact, or even like possible avoidance. If you're a partner, lover, friend or carer of someone during treatment, I implore you, I beg you, to offer them touch. Treatment is damaging and also detaching. We need the treatment, yes, but we also need care, to feel connected to ourselves and to those around us. Don't be afraid of us, be cautious and curious with us. Think of it as getting into 'ask first' mode.

For simple touch, a peck on the lips or cheek? It's okay! We are not radioactive, we won't give you cancer and we won't break, if we all just take a little care. How do we know what to do or what not to do? We ask.

How to say it out loud.

- "Would you like me to take your hand?"
- "Is there any way you might like some loving/comforting touch right now?"
- "Would you like a hug?"
- "I'd love a cuddle; how does that sound to you?"
- "I'd love to connect with you, are there any sore spots I should avoid if I went in for a cuddle?"
- "I'd love to connect with you right now, is there a form of touch you would like?" (Arm around the shoulder, hand holding, hug from behind, foot massage and more.)
- "I love you and want to offer you affection, is there anything that would comfort you at the moment?"

- "I miss you, but I'm worried I'll hurt you if I squeeze you too hard. Is there a way I can snuggle into you?"
- "I'm wanting to show you love and affection, such as a kiss on the lips or cheek, how do you feel about that?"
- "I'm checking you out right now, fancy a kiss?"

If you're being made an offer of connection and it's not a good time? A simple, "thank you, but I'm not quite up for it at the moment" is perfect. Even if the person receiving this offer is not up for it right then, you're showing love, care, concern for their well-being and the desire to remain connected. It means the world.

Not in the mood?

Whether you're the person with cancer or the partner of, there will be times when you don't feel like being intimate with others, that is fine, that is normal, that is understandable. There will also be times when you feel like connecting somehow, but aren't sure how. There are lots of places to start: Get in the bath and relax or wrap yourself in blankets with a hot-water bottle, maybe touch your body, snuggle a pet with your favourite film, ask the person you're with to intertwine your legs while you both sit on the couch or lean into their chest. During treatments, you're not going to want intimacy or touch all of the time, so feel free to let loved ones know how you're feeling and speak up in the moments it seems plausible. If you do receive an offer of intimacy and connection and you're not up for it? Remember, that's okay, that's fine, that's normal. But also remember to say thanks for the offer and be kind when you say no thanks, because you want the offers to keep coming!

How to say it out loud.

- "Thank you, that sounds amazing, it's not the best moment, can we see how I'm going later?" (Or tomorrow, or after lunch)
- "Thanks, I'm feeling quite nauseous/tired/some pain, for the moment I need to sit still, can we maybe connect later or another day?"
- "I'm really not feeling well, I'd like to sit alone for a while. Thank you so much for offering a cuddle, rain-check?"
- "I'd love to kiss you, but my mouth is a bit sore at

the moment, would you like some soft neck touch instead?"

- "I'd love a hug, thank you, could you be careful around my arm? It's a bit sore."
- "I don't think I'm up for a hug right now, would you like to hold my hand?"
- "I'm pretty low on energy at the moment, but something soft and gentle would be lovely, like a snuggle?"
- Or if you're ADHD and ridiculously blunt like me "Thanks for the offer of a kiss, I'm currently trying not to vomit in my mouth, so will need to rain-check" (we both had a giggle at that).

To those undergoing treatments, if you feel your partner/lover/friend is avoiding you, unattracted to you and doesn't want to touch you? They may just be thinking they are protecting you, avoiding potentially hurting you or feel like they're pestering/pressuring you, so are pulling away. Be the one to communicate and offer a connection. Offer to snuggle, offer to touch their back while they're standing next to you, ask for a long hug hello, it guides them, and can lead to further connections. It meant the world to me, having my hand held and legs entwined on the couch with a cup of tea and chats. Simple things like that were so important, and I know is/was to others during treatments.

11. FOR MY FELLOW RAINBOW-FLAGGERS

For people in the LGBTQIA+ community, medical institutions can be very difficult. I remember sitting in the chemo-chair with my then partner holding my hand. The nurse approached and looked at us holding hands, then looking at her said "oh, isn't that sweet you're such good *friends*". I know the nurse meant well, but it was devaluing to me and my partner. I did not feel like I was seen as a person, nor my partner respected. I also did not have the energy to continually educate everyone around me all day every day and advocate for who I am and for others. It's exhausting and with cancer, I didn't have it in me. So, I withdrew and I became reluctant to share my personal story with most clinicians. This is particularly important for people with cancers such as prostate, testicular, cervix, ovaries or breast (just to name a few), as these cancers are *very* gendered. Due to this people can isolate themselves from the supports that are out there as they may feel unwelcome or unseen. Speaking personally, the 'sisterhood' is very strong in breast cancer and as a non-binary person, was difficult to ignore. I avoided so many (pretty much all) support networks due to this as I did not feel welcome. If you're someone who resonates with this, if you belong to communities that are marginalised, I ask you to reach out. Reach out to that one person on your treating team you can have an honest, non-shaming conversation with. Reach out to the nurse asking for any resources the hospital knows of that are accessible and inclusive. Reach out to a friend, to find a cancer support group near you or online that is gender aware, recognises pronouns, alternative relationship models, and partnerships that are not only heterosexual. They are out there, but you may need help finding them. Feeling safe and supported is everything.

RESOURCES

Because there's limited work on sexuality and cancer and well, actual realistic and accessible sexuality education in general, resources can be hard to find. So, here are some, of varied mediums depending on what suits you best.

The 'A Better Normal' mini-book series

Available globally on Amazon in paperback or eBook format, you can search by author 'Tess Devèze' or by book title.

If you're needing support, practical solutions and guidance on more specific side-effects, or looking for help regarding a specific treatment, the 'A Better Normal' mini-book series covers quite a range.

Books in the 'A Better Normal' mini-book series are:

- 'A Better Normal for **Libido**; Your Guide to Rediscovering Intimacy After Cancer'
- 'A Better Normal for **Vaginal Dryness & Pain**; Your Guide to Rediscovering Intimacy After Cancer'
- 'A Better Normal for **Body Confidence**; Your Guide to Rediscovering Intimacy After Cancer'

- 'A Better Normal for **Chemotherapy**; Your Guide to Rediscovering Intimacy After Cancer'
- 'A Better Normal for **Hormone Therapy**; Your Guide to Rediscovering Intimacy After Cancer'
- 'A Better Normal for **Fatigue**; Your Guide to Rediscovering Intimacy After Cancer'
- 'A Better Normal for **Changes in Erection**; Your Guide to Rediscovering Intimacy After Cancer'
- 'A Better Normal for **Radiotherapy**; Your Guide to Rediscovering Intimacy After Cancer'
- 'A Better Normal for **Pain**; Your Guide to Rediscovering Intimacy After Cancer'

The all-in-one resource, 'A Better Normal; Your Guide to Rediscovering Intimacy After Cancer'

Available globally on Amazon in paperback or eBook, you can search via author 'Tess Devèze' or by book title.

If you liked the information in this book, but feel you need guidance on more, the book 'A Better Normal; Your Guide to Rediscovering Intimacy After Cancer' has all of the information included in the entire mini-book series and more. It's your one stop shop for everything you need to know about sexuality and cancer, in the one book.

Vulva Pleasure Masterclass

(connectable.podia.com/vulva-masterclass)

For anyone with a vulva who is experiencing pain and dryness, or is experiencing loss of sensation, pleasure, arousal and orgasm. This online Masterclass teaches vulva massage, which can be done on yourself or with a partner. Through massage and neurological concepts, things like arousal and pleasure can be recovered while helping heal tissues through increasing blood-flow with massage. This Masterclass is also suitable for people with vaginismus and vulvodynia.

Penis Pleasure Masterclass

(connectable.podia.com/penis-pleasure)

For anyone with a penis who is experiencing changes in erection and orgasm, or is experiencing loss of sensation, function and pleasure. This online Masterclass teaches soft penis massage, which can be done on yourself or with a partner. Through massage and neurological concepts, things like sensation and pleasure can be recovered while helping recover erectile function through increasing blood-flow with massage. This Masterclass is particularly beneficial for people post prostatectomy.

A libido and intimacy recovery program for couples 'Connection & Cancer: Reclaim Your Intimacy & Desire'. (connectable.podia.com/libido-after-cancer)

If the libido information in this book made sense, but you would like personal support through the exact process of *how* to recover your pleasure, intimacy and libido, then this is for you. It's with me online guiding you every step of the way, and is done in the privacy of your own home. Filled with information, fun and practical solutions that I take you through for libido recovery. The people who I've worked with in this program are having life-changing results. It's an absolute honour to guide people to recover what they felt was lost forever.

'ConnectAble Therapies' (connectabletherapies.com) For consultations and further resources on sex, intimacy & cancer.

Facebook global support group: *'Intimacy and Cancer'*. This group is for any cancer, any gender and is a very supportive space.

Instagram '@connectable_therapies', where I regularly share helpful information.

YouTube Channel on sex, intimacy & cancer: type *"Intimacy and Cancer CHANNEL"* to find it.

If you prefer video formats over reading (as cancer-brain & reading don't go well together), this YouTube Channel is filled with short videos discussing all things sex, intimacy and cancer.

'ConnectAble Courses' (connectable.podia.com)

A site of intimacy and cancer online courses for sexual recovery. Including the Masterclasses, libido recovery program and webinar mentioned here.

Intimacy & Cancer Information Webinar

(connectable.podia.com/webinar-intimacyaftercancer)

A free information webinar discussing the impacts cancer treatments have on intimacy and sexuality. It has a particular focus on libido and how it can be recovered.

Other amazing resources:

'A Touchy Subject' (atouchysubject.com)

For people with prostate cancer or experiencing changes in erection. Victoria Cullen is *the* person to go to, about sexuality and intimacy post a prostate cancer diagnosis. She also has a YouTube channel and through her website access to free resources and rehabilitation programs.

'The Art of The Hook Up' (artofthehookup.com)
This site from dating expert and communication extraordinaire is by Georgie Wolf. Not cancer specific, but incredibly on-point and with relative information for anyone struggling with the dating scene. She has podcasts, blogs, eBooks and more. She's also a workshop facilitator and a bit of a superstar here in Australia!

'Curious Creatures' (curiouscreatures.biz)
For online workshops and much more education on self-development and sexuality. They provide articles, podcasts and streamable workshops which are all very practical and very accessible. I have the privilege to work for this company, their work is changing lives.

'Bump'n Joystick' (getbumpn.com)
An intimacy aid designed for people with impaired upper

limb and fine-motor function. Suitable for all genders and is flexible to varied body shapes. This toy was designed by the global disability and OT community, and it's pretty incredible.

'The Ziggy' (luddi.co)

Another intimacy aid designed for people with limited upper limb and intact fine-motor function. Designed by the disability community and healthcare professionals, this is a multi-purpose vibrator for all genders. It's also able to be used while in a wheelchair, so is a wonderfully accessible item.

Pelvic and sexual health osteopath

For those who live in Melbourne, Australia, we have one of the top pelvic health osteopaths you'll ever find. Dr Andrew Carr from the *'Whole Being Health Collective'* is referred to as *'the body whisperer'* in clinical and sexual health circles. He works with the entire body, however has expertise and clinical focus on pelvic and sexual health. In particular, people experiencing pelvic pain including after treatments, vaginismus, atrophy and is trauma informed.

If you're not located in Melbourne, there are pelvic

floor osteopaths, physiotherapists and OTs all over the world. Simply search online "Pelvic floor osteopath/physio/OT (insert the name of your city/town here)". You'll find someone near you.

Support groups in your area

If you search in google "Cancer Support (insert city/town where you live here)", there should be a list of businesses and companies that have programs near you. Some online or in person. They mightn't be sexuality specific, but there is always opportunity for discussions and learning.

ACKNOWLEDGEMENTS

For anyone and everyone out there affected by cancer, this book is for you. There can be so much to consider, to have to endure, to have to keep track of, that many parts of life take a back seat. Thank you for caring about your intimacy and connections during such a time, be it connections with yourself or with others. I hope you're supported and I truly hope there is something in this book for you.

I'm forever grateful to my clients and the thousands I support online who so openly and vulnerably share their struggles, and also their triumphs with me. This book would not exist without you. I'm inspired and amazed by you all, daily.

Thank you, to my partners and carers over the years Rog, Robi and Kane, my family and my global network of friends. There were some very dark places during treatments and you all got me through. To my booby buddies (my breast care nurses) Claire & Monique, you're my angels. Ricky Dick my oncologist - you're simply the best (Tina Turner style!) and to my RADelaidies.

Lastly, to acknowledge the incredible ethics, values and

approaches to sexuality and communication from Roger Butler at Curious Creatures (and their generosity with sharing their content with me), the occupational therapy & sexuality community (yeah OT-siggers!) and the revolutionary perspectives and therapeutic trainings I received from Deej & Uma, at the Institute of Somatic Sexology (ISS).

ABOUT THE AUTHOR

Tess Devèze is an occupational therapist (OT) having completed their bachelor degree in Melbourne Australia, founding ConnectAble Therapies, a community sexuality OT and sexology clinic focussing on sexuality and intimacy for people with neurological conditions, cancer, chronic illness and disability. They have also completed certification and trainings via the Institute of Somatic Sexology. Alongside being a sexuality OT, Tess is also a sexuality educator & workshop facilitator, and has facilitated and educated thousands of people in the topics of communication, consent, sexuality, pleasure and relationship dynamics for nearing a decade. Tess founded the global online initiative 'Intimacy and Cancer', an online support space for people of all cancers and genders to access sexual support.

As a non-binary, queer, disabled person living with cancer, Tess's work is inclusive and advocates for sexual rights for disabled, neurodivergent, gender queer/diverse and LGBTQIA+, communities, which they proudly belong to.

Tess was diagnosed with stage 3 breast cancer at the age of 36 and is still undergoing treatments.

Find them at www.connectabletherapies.com

DID YOU ENJOY THE BOOK?

As an independent author, my work survives through your support. There are so many people affected by cancer, suffering in silence. With each review or word-of-mouth recommendation you make, we can reach the many out there who are struggling and need support.

Please leave a review by visiting where you purchased this book. It's just 1 minute of your time, but could be the thing that helps this reach someone who needs it, someone who needs a better normal too.

Got feedback? Please leave a review! Plus, I'd love to hear from you. You can reach me via email at tess@connectabletherapies.com or via Instagram @connectable_therapies.